keeping life simple

keeping life simple

380 TIPS & IDEAS

KAREN LEVINE

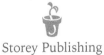

Storey Publishing

The mission of Storey Publishing is to serve our customers by publishing practical information that encourages personal independence in harmony with the environment.

Cover and text design by Carol Jessop
Cover photo courtesy of Polywoodinc.com
Copyright © 2004 Storey Publishing, LLC

The information in this book is true and complete to the best of our knowledge. All recommendations are made without guarantee on the part of the author or Storey Publishing. The author and publisher disclaim any liability in connection with the use of this information. For additional information please contact Storey Publishing, 210 MASS MoCA Way, North Adams, MA 01247.

Storey books are available for special premium and promotional uses and for customized editions. For further information, please call 1-800-793-9396.

Printed in the United States by Von Hoffmann
10 9 8 7 6 5 4 3 2 1

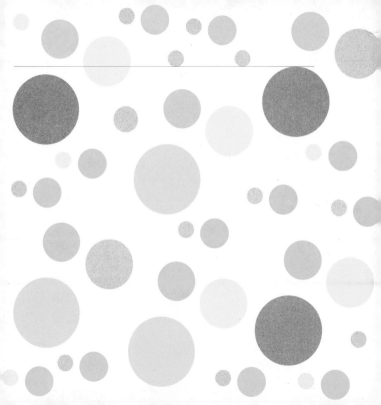

FOR MOST OF US EACH DAY IS PACKED and life can feel pretty cluttered. How do people who feel they are doing more/earning more/getting more but enjoying it all less manage to turn things around and focus on building more satisfying lives? How do we sort through all the "stuff" and find the meaning that we long for? How can we simplify and enhance our lives?

This book attempts to answer those questions on two levels. On a pragmatic level, with tips and hints, and on an aesthetic level with things you can do to simplify, and thereby enhance, your life. Different people find satisfaction in different ways. This idea might seem obvious, but you'd be surprised by how many people devote their energies to trying to be happy in a prescribed way, rather than to trying to determine what it is that really makes them happy. The key, of course, is to figure out what your idea of heaven is, and to simplify your life so that you can get as close to it as possible. How do you accomplish that? **READ ON...**

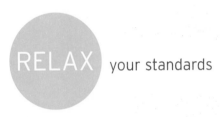

RELAX your standards

Take time to figure out

what you find most

SATISFYING.

CREATE TIME for the

things you care about, whether it is

daily exercise or 30 minutes with a

good book.

ENJOY

what's in front
of you.

There is a value in having a long-range perspective on life, but there is also a value in being able to live in the moment.

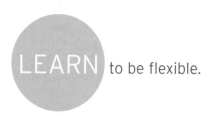

LEARN to be flexible.

Rigidity is the hobgoblin of

an unsatisfying life.

CHANGE ... every once in a

while you need to shake things up

and surprise everyone, including

yourself.

Surprise your kids by not reacting

to them the way they

think you will. BEND.

QUESTION yourself every time you "take a stand." There are many stands worth taking, but there are also stands that have lost their significance.

The fine line between being flexible,

being wishy-washy, and being rigid

is worth EXPLORING!

What activities and things are you

able to live without?

Remember, you always have the

capacity to make CHOICES.

ASK yourself how much time

you spend picking out clothing; put-

ting on makeup; making breakfast

(for yourself and for others); pack-

ing lunches; looking for your keys.

CREATE pleasurable experi-

ences. Draw yourself a bath with

wonderful oils, light a dozen candles,

turn on some soft music, and

settle in for an hour.

There are things we do that aren't really pleasurable but are, nonetheless, quite satisfying. Take the time to think about what it is you enjoy doing, and what it is that gives you a sense of satisfaction.

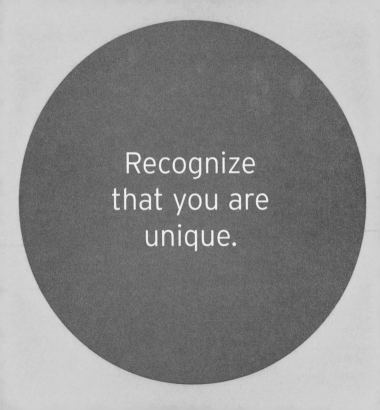

Recognize
that you are
unique.

There are no bonus points in life for

suffering through what other people

say you should ENJOY.

AVOID the hectic pace of the

supermarket by doing your grocery

shopping at a local store.

SPEND the most time on the

activities that give you the greatest

pleasure or satisfaction.

You may have more control over

your time than you think.

Even before you can put your hands

into the earth to dig a garden you

may feel the need to buy a lot of

specialty items. DON'T.

CURL UP in a comfortable

chair and listen to your

favorite music.

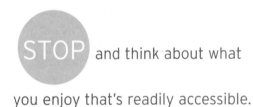 **STOP** and think about what you enjoy that's readily accessible.

Pour yourself some tea, coffee, hot

chocolate, wine – whatever you like

– and enjoy what you're about to

READ.

MAKE your bedroom inviting,

serene, and maybe even sensual.

Take a moment to make your bed

in the morning.

KEEP a pad and pencil near your

bed. You may wake up from a dream

that is well worth writing down!

LOOK UP

and notice a
spectacular,
inspiring night sky.

Try treating the Sabbath as a true day of rest. Turn on your answering machine, go for a walk or a bike ride, play some non-electronic games with your family, sing, make music, or read the entire newspaper cover to cover.

TAKE a vacation without going anywhere. By the end of the vacation you should be able to say, "Now I remember why I live where I do."

There are probably hikes in your

area that culminate with a great

view. Ask for a book on local hikes

at your LIBRARY.

IF you live in an area that experiences real winters, buy yourself a set of flannel sheets. You'll begin to eagerly anticipate crawling into bed at about 4:00 P.M.

If you've got a fireplace,

USE IT.

MAKE a campfire in your back-

yard on a beautiful summer night.

Bake bread. Get your hands into the dough, work out some frustrations, watch it rise, punch it down, and then relax and enjoy the sweet smell while it BAKES.

GIVE yourself a half hour at the end of the day to unwind by doing whatever feels relaxing to you: reading, listening to music, meditating, and so on.

Get a few books about your feath-

ered friends and the homes they

build for themselves. Then look

around OUTSIDE.

SUPPORT public radio. For

whatever you're inclined to give

you'll get countless hours of won-

derful news and entertaining

programming. Do it!

If you enjoy wind chimes, buy a really good set. You don't want to hear a lot of clunking noises every time the wind blows.

REFRESH an old dresser or

chair with stencils, marbleizing,

sponging, or texturing with paint.

BUY yourself some flowers.

There's nothing so satisfying as getting

a great bargain. Tag sales, thrift shops,

end-of-season sales, used sporting

equipment stores, newspaper ads, and

friends who are looking to dump

some stuff . . . that's where you begin.

SPLURGE a little on

something you've always wanted.

TRY a tin of exotic imported tea.

When you're finished with the tea,

the handsome tin will make a useful

receptacle.

REMEMBER the old adage:

"The past is history, the future a

mystery, but today is a gift, which is

why it is called the Present."

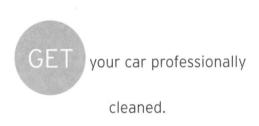 your car professionally

cleaned.

TAKE five minutes to relax your

back, neck, and facial muscles.

The next time you are on a long car

trip by yourself write a song and

sing it out loud.

Take a few massage classes with

your partner or a good friend, and

then do it for each other.

FIND something that appeals to

your sense of fancy that's also

inexpensive, and begin a collection.

FORGET about those baby bathtubs and run a nice deep tub for yourself and your little one. Sit with your knees up and put your baby on your tummy.

Help yourself to relax by practicing square breathing. BREATHE in to the count of four, hold it for the count of four, exhale for the count of four and pause for the count of four. Now do it all again . . . and again . . . and again . . . BREATHE in to the count of four, hold it for the count of four, exhale for the count of four and pause for the count of four. Now do it all again . . . and again . . . and again.

WHEN someone new moves onto your block, make it a point to go over and say hello.

KEEP a cheap pair of lawn chairs

in the trunk of your car. You never

know when you'll pass a beautiful

meadow or a wonderful old grave-

yard that beckons you to come and

sit for a while.

Plan an afternoon with your children

on an "Adventure into the Unknown."

Think of three or four places that

they've never been. Places to think

about include: airports, tall office build-

ings, parks, factories, and museums.

Take your children on a trip to see where you lived when you were a KID.

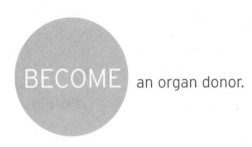 an organ donor.

CHECK out books on tape from

your public library for the car trip to

and from work.

Exchange a gift that doesn't

delight YOU.

TRY out the music your parents

listened to when they were your

age. You may have a wonderful sur-

prise in store!

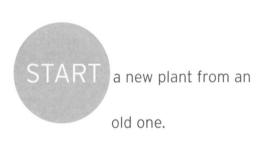

START a new plant from an

old one.

WOOD-BURNING saunas

don't cost much to build, and the

psychic benefits are enormous.

READ aloud to children, your own or someone else's. Many elementary schools welcome volunteers.

The art of art, the glory of expression and the sunshine of the light of letters, is simplicity.

WALT WHITMAN (1819-1892)

LISTEN. It's easy to fall into

the habit of listening to what other

people have to say only so you can

come up with a response.

Pot a few Paper White narcissus

bulbs in gravel or soil and put them

in a cool dark place for a few weeks.

Then bring them into the light and

water sparingly until shoots appear.

You'll have a fabulous narcissus

bloom in the middle of the winter.

Take your dog for a good long

WALK.

Listen to the sounds around you

when you go for a walk.

ENJOY your sense of smell.

Smell the bread baking, the coffee,

the grass, the baby's neck, and any-

thing else that makes you feel good.

REFLECT on
what you have to
be grateful about.

IF you've spent the last twenty-five

years or so avoiding your college or

high school reunion, rethink it.

Take a ten minute walk for no

purpose other than being

OUTSIDE.

TRY keeping a journal. It will feel

luxurious while you're doing it, as

well as in the years to come.

PRESS some flowers.

Take pleasure in your garden

all year long.

LEARN about the area in which you live. Start with your local library or historical society or talk to an old-timer.

TAKE a bath with some wonder-

fully fragrant essential oils and a

dozen votive candles.

Throw your towels or terry robe in

the dryer before you get into the

tub and ask someone to bring them

to you when you're ready to get out.

Heated towels. MMMM!

VISIT the neighborhood in

which you grew up.

ENJOY your snow days.

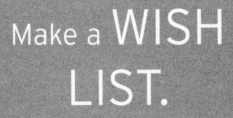

Make a WISH LIST.

SLOW DOWN...

even if you're in a hurry.

THINK about the activities that

give you the most pleasure.

Sometimes, if you really allow your-

self to get lost in the thought, it's

almost as good as being there.

STEP outside before you're

ready to go to bed and look up at

the starry sky.

Pull over to the side of the road

and watch the SUN SET.

We tend to think of time as some-

thing that must be used produc-

tively. It's also important to take

time to DO NOTHING.

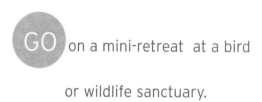 **GO** on a mini-retreat at a bird

or wildlife sanctuary.

GO to your local library and check

out some CDs that offer a kind of

music you don't ordinarily hear.

GIVE someone an unexpected gift.

MEET your child's school bus on

a stormy day with flowers for the

driver.

Think of things that you've always

done the same way and try, instead,

to wander down an alternate path.

97

INDULGE yourself with an

hour of doing nothing but listening

to your favorite music.

Find some quiet time to think . . .

about where you are in life, about

your goals, about your disappoint-

ments, and so on. Insight can be

very curative and energizing, but it

requires THOUGHT.

GIVE yourself a small task that

you know you will be able to begin

and complete in a satisfying way.

Pick a small cabinet to clean out or

organize a drawer.

Allow yourself the

satisfaction of getting a job done.

BUY a few scented geraniums for your home. They're easy to care for, and when you brush their leaves they release wonderful fragrances of mint, lemon, rose, orange, nutmeg, and more.

KEEP downtime sacred and

don't feel guilty about it.

The least of things with a meaning is worth more in life than the greatest of things without it.

CARL JUNG (1875-1961)

EVEN if you don't meditate, you

can practice one of meditation's most

valuable lessons: Do only what you

are doing, be only where you are.

Stop mowing your lawn and plant a meadow.

PLANT a cutting garden near

enough to the house for you to step

out every day and cut some fresh

flowers.

MAKE an indoor winter herb garden. Best choices for an indoor garden include basil, bay, chives, mint, parsley, and thyme.

SHARE your plants. Part of the

joy of gardening is its conviviality.

MAKE COMPOST.

It's good for the earth and means

less smelly garbage for you to haul

to the dump.

RIDE a bicycle to work or to

do an errand.

If you've been avoiding your yearly

physical exam, chances are you're

worried about something. The worry

will show itself one way or another.

Get the physical and breathe a sigh

of RELIEF.

TRY not to sit for more than

thirty minutes at a time without

taking a break – get up and stretch

for five minutes.

INSTEAD of going to the gym,

walk with a friend.

Avoid using a doctor with whom you don't feel entirely comfortable. If your doctor is not a person with whom you can have a relaxed conversation about your health, she isn't the doctor for you.

RUN up a flight of stairs instead

of using the elevator.

Are you getting all the sleep you need? Sleep triggers a growth hormone to renew tissues, form new red blood cells, and promote bone formation. Best of all it enables you to DREAM.

GIVE yourself a regular bedtime

and allow yourself a good half hour

to get ready.

Before you go to sleep at night, lie in bed and try this relaxation exercise; begin by saying "Relax my toes," and make a conscious effort to relax them, continue all the way up to your forehead. Don't miss any area . . . they're probably all filled with tension.

GET a better night's sleep –

replace your box spring and mattress

if they are eight to ten years old.

It is vain to say human beings ought to be satisfied with tranquility: They must have action; and they will make it if they cannot find it.

CHARLOTTE BRONTÉ (1816–1855)

Don't exercise too close to bedtime.

It can be too stimulating and inter-

fere with your SLEEP.

IF you wake up in the middle of the night, anxious about all that awaits you in the day to come, get up and write a list for yourself. There! It's on paper. Now go back to sleep.

WARM milk is a natural tran-

quilizer and calcium helps you relax.

Try a glass at night before you go

to bed.

SOOTHE your tired eyes. Put two wet tea bags in the freezer for a couple of minutes while you gently rub some cooking oil over your eyelids. Take the tea bags out and put them on your lids for about fifteen minutes.

MAKE AND KEEP

a dinner date with your "significant

other" at least once a month.

TAKE up a new hobby with your partner, something that interests both of you. Join a choir; take a computer or cooking class; study Chinese; take up bird watching, ballroom dancing, or bowling.

FIND time to spend with friends – even if it's just an hour of sipping tea and talking.

WHEN you walk into the house

at the end of the day, set aside

some time for your children that will

be exclusively theirs.

IF you have trouble getting along with your in-laws, remind yourself that they must have done some-thing right . . . after all, they man-aged to turn out the person with whom you are spending your life.

Never make public statements, con-

frontations, or write anything down

in the heat of PASSION.

SHARE a good feeling you have

with your kids, your spouse, your

friends, and your co-workers.

NETWORKING is as simple

as connecting with people to whom

you might be helpful and who might

be helpful to you.

WRITE a letter to a friend or

family member.

CREATE TIME for intimacy

with your partner. Get into bed an

hour early and you'll have time to

enjoy each other . . . and remember

how nice that is.

JOIN a local theater group or, if

you're not interested in participat-

ing, go to a performance.

FIND something you want to

learn about and become an

expert on it.

USE your commuting time to

learn a foreign language.

DANCE with someone you like.

REVISIT the religion you

grew up with.

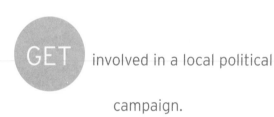 involved in a local political

campaign.

IF you love to cook good food why

not find some other people who

share your passion and get together

once a month.

EVERY NEW YEAR'S I write a long letter to a friend telling her about my year. Other than that letter we rarely talk, but the annual communication has become important to us both. This year she wrote, "I have kept your letters for the last sixteen years and as I read them now they come together, in a very beautiful way, to make a life. THANK YOU."

FIND OUT what's growing in

your backyard.

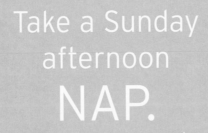

Take a Sunday afternoon NAP.

Learn the Japanese art of origami.

KNITTING really is a simple pleasure . . . a sort of mantra for your fingers with a wonderful gift at the end!

THINK about a book that you

absolutely loved when you were in

college, and reread it.

START an online reading group

with long-distance friends.

DECIDE not to read the book

you've been carrying for months in

your purse or in the car. Put it away

and choose something else.

IF there's one near you,

join a CSA farm. Community

supported agriculture is good

for everybody.

The price we pay for the complexity of life is too high. When you think of all the effort you have to put in . . . to alter even the slightest bit of behavior in this strange world we call social life, you are left pining for the straightforwardness of primitive peoples and their physical work.

JEAN BAUDRILLARD (1929–)

DROP out of one committee or evening meeting and dedicate that time to family activities.

WHEN you put your children to

bed, don't ask them how their day

was. Instead, ask them what the

best part of their day was.

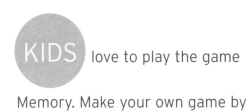 **KIDS** love to play the game

Memory. Make your own game by

ordering double photos.

Keep a scrapbook for your child that includes the front page of the newspaper on the day of his/her birthday every year.

MAKE

water balloons
on a hot summer
day.

Spend an evening together with

your family playing Scrabble,

Monopoly, Chess, Checkers, or

PARCHEESI.

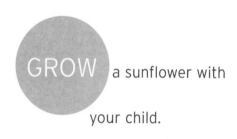

GROW a sunflower with your child.

Roast marshmallows over a candle.

FRAME and hang your

children's artistic endeavors.

TALK to your oldest living rela-

tive about his or her childhood mem-

ories and record the conversation.

Research your

FAMILY TREE.

I adore simple pleasures. They are the last refuge of the complex.

Oscar Wilde (1854–1900)

GO APPLE PICKING.

SEND flowers to a good friend

for no special reason.

CREATE
your own
unexpected
celebrations.

OFFER to drive a homebound

person to visit family for Christmas.

Sing Christmas carols at a

NURSING HOME.

THIS Thanksgiving, double up on

your cooking and bring a meal to

someone who wouldn't otherwise

have it.

Tell your kids how you celebrated

things when you were YOUNG.

THINK of ways to celebrate

Christmas, Passover, birthdays,

Kwanzaa, that leave you and your

family feeling renewed.

If you have children who find it a

terrible chore to dress up for a holi-

day, try letting go of this require-

ment and allowing everyone to

dress as they PLEASE.

AT our happiest moments we can

take a moment to think about how

difficult life can be.

Allow for some downtime during the

busy holiday SEASON.

DON'T become trapped by

obligation during the holidays.

If sending holiday cards is a source

of frustration and guilt, simply stop.

IF you've hosted the traditional family Christmas, Chanukah, Easter, or Passover for the last ten years, think about taking a year off and finding a place to be the guest!

Share your holiday traditions.

CONSIDER using a disposable

roasting pan for your turkey.

EMPTY a jar or more of marinated artichoke hearts into a food processor for the world's easiest dip. Add to taste lemon juice, fresh garlic, and olive oil. Puree. Perfect for crusty bread or crudité.

Throw a party for a friend on a special BIRTHDAY.

ANY cake looks special when it's decorated with curls of choco-late, and they're very easy to make. Scrape a chocolate bar with a vegetable peeler and heap shavings on top.

PICK UP GIFTS whenever

you see something you think some-

one would like, rather than wait for

the occasion.

Don't bake a cake if it ends up being

a chore. There are great mixes and

even better BAKERIES!

Make a contribution in someone's

name instead of giving a GIFT.

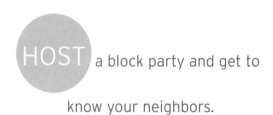 **HOST** a block party and get to know your neighbors.

KEEP a few generic children's toys or games on hand. You'll always have something ready for a birthday gift.

ALWAYS use in-store

gift wrapping services.

KEEP gift-wrapping paper, ribbons, a pair of scissors, and a roll of tape in a big box, so that whenever you go to wrap a gift you have what you need on hand.

LET your children know that a gift need not be an object.

Don't over-invite when it comes to

your kid's birthday PARTY.

HAVE a natural scavenger hunt for a child's birthday party. Let kids search for worms, pinecones, acorns, different-colored rocks, and flowers.

GIVE the gift of babysitting.

The aspects of things that are most important for us are hidden because of their simplicity and familiarity.

LUDWIG WITTGENSTEIN (1889–1951)

HAVE THE WEDDING

YOU WANT.

LOVE means not having

to spend a fortune on an

anniversary gift.

BUY a pretty, small notebook;
over the course of the year, make a
note of the times your lover does
something to remind you of why you
got together in the first place. By
the end of the year the notebook
will make the perfect Valentine's
Day gift.

CELEBRATE St. Patrick's

Day. You don't have to be Irish to

enjoy a holiday in March.

DURING the eight days of

Passover consider donating the

foods you are not permitted to eat.

Have a corn-on-the-cob dinner for

LABOR DAY.

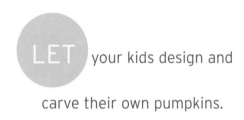 **LET** your kids design and carve their own pumpkins.

Light a menorah for each member

of the family during Chanukah.

One week before Christmas have a big gathering and spend the day baking dozens of cookies. When you're all done, divide up the varieties and everyone will have an ample share of Christmas cookies.

Make a recording of your family

caroling TOGETHER.

IF your Christmas tree lights are

all tangled, get new ones.

Show your kids
how to make snow
ANGELS.

POT an amaryllis bulb and you'll have an absolute show-stopper centerpiece for the holiday table.

Give your Christmas tree a new look. DECORATE it with things found in nature: pinecones, bird nests, seashells, bittersweet, moss. It's free, and you'll be amazed how BEAUTIFUL it is.

DON'T WAIT

for the holiday season to start

buying Christmas presents.

MAKE it a rule to order double

sets of photographs.

I have learned to have very modest goals for society and myself, things like clean air, green grass, children with bright eyes, not being pushed around, useful work that suits one's abilities, plain tasty food . . .

PAUL GOODMAN (1911–1972)

EVERY once in a while give

yourself a mental health day . . . a

"holiday" for no reason other than

the fact that you deserve it.

"THINNING OUT"

applies not only to stuff but to

activities and sometimes people.

Don't do something simply because

you didn't know how to say "no."

IF you feel that you don't have time to complete things, break the job into smaller units.

READ A
SHORT STORY.

DETERMINE exactly what is

most important to accomplish in any

given day.

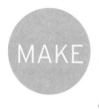 **MAKE** a list you know you can

accomplish.

START your to-do list with something quick and easy so you can cross off several "to do" items from your list right away!

STOP
over-scheduling
your children.

PUT your television in a closet

for a month.

Use your lunch time to regroup.

Find a quiet space to meditate in,

sit outside and read, or take a long,

VIGOROUS WALK.

CONSIDER hiring someone to

help you clean your house.

MAKE an effort to break the habit of being late. It causes more stress to be late than it does to be a little early.

KEEP only one calendar

or date book, and keep it with you

at all times.

Plan some aspects of your days so

that they are set and not open to

NEGOTIATION.

HAVE YOUR KIDS
PICK OUT THEIR
WARDROBES FOR
THE WEEK ON
SUNDAY NIGHT.

KEEP pocket change in a bowl near the door so you have change when you need it . . . for calls from pay phones, school lunches, tolls for bridges, and the like.

SET YOUR ALARM

for a half-hour early every morning

and think of that time as all yours.

SET CERTAIN TIMES

of the day during which you simply

don't answer the phone.

GET RID of your answering

machine or voice mail. You'll never

have to "return" a call again.

CONSIDER dropping call-waiting from your phone service. It is annoying to you and to the person you're speaking with.

You must learn to be still in the midst of activity and to be vibrantly alive in repose.

INDIRA GANDHI (1917–1984)

Group your errands and shopping so

that you don't spend time retracing

your steps.

SOME errands are fun with children in tow, but others are nearly impossible. Learn to distinguish.

USE automatic services for your

banking and bill paying.

GIVE yourself time every now

and then to have a weekend

with no plans.

KEEP an enjoyable activity in

mind for when you have unexpected

time. Use that time as a gift to your-

self if your dental appointment has

been canceled or a business lunch

falls through.

SPEND
time with people
you like.

Don't give up entertaining because

it's too much work. Do it differently.

DEVELOP traditions that

make you and your family feel

relaxed and united.

ALLOW open time in your

schedule to deal with unexpected

events that you can't anticipate.

THINK about the possibility of

you or your spouse downshifting to

part-time. You may need the time

more than the income.

BECOME a volunteer for

something you care about.

DON'T over-commit yourself.

Start out with a small commitment

and build up.

Are you working to support a

lifestyle that isn't all that important

or SATISFYING?

Make a distinction between the

things that you need and the things

that you simply DESIRE.

Simplicity, simplicity, simplicity! I say, let your affairs be as two or three, and not a hundred or a thousand; instead of a million count half a dozen, and keep your accounts on your thumb-nail.

HENRY DAVID THOREAU (1817–1862)

LIVE BELOW YOUR MEANS.

Use a charge card that must be paid

in its entirety every month.

CANCEL a subscription to a

magazine that you don't really have

time to read.

Buy more than one of the things

you always NEED.

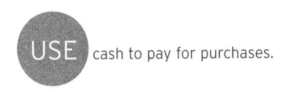 cash to pay for purchases.

EAT WHAT'S IN
SEASON.
EAT WHAT'S LOCAL.

CONVENIENCE foods

aren't always that convenient and

they always cost more.

KEEP a folder for coupons in

your car.

JOIN A FOOD CO-OP.

THINK TWICE before

buying something new.

Subdue your appetites, my dears, and you've conquered human nature.

CHARLES DICKENS (1812–1870)

Bring your lunch to work.

THE hidden expense of shopping by mail is handling and postage charges. You can reduce this expense by pooling orders with friends and taking advantage of reduced shipping offers.

REFRAIN from shopping as a

form of entertainment.

LIMIT your wardrobe to a few

colors that go well together.

GIVEN the choice between buy-

ing a few cheap things or one high-

quality item, buy the single treasure.

Buy fewer pairs of shoes and buy

good ones.

Always buy
clothes that fit.

MAKE believe you're moving

and go through your house room by

room – pruning clutter ruthlessly.

BE HONEST with yourself

about your own personal tolerance

for clutter.

SORT things out as soon as

they come into your home, or the

moment you are finished with them.

Find a place to put your mail every

day and never deviate from it.

Try having a little less of everything.

NEVER leave a room without

picking up something that needs to

be put away.

The art of being wise is the art of knowing what to overlook.

GO through your pantry and refrigerator and put all the food you never use but have somehow acquired (anchovies, sardines, oatmeal, cardamom, whatever) in a large bag. Give it to a food pantry or throw it away.

GET RID of duplicate gadgets.

You don't need three vegetable

peelers and four soufflé dishes.

CLEAR OUT your medicine

chest regularly and toss what you

don't use.

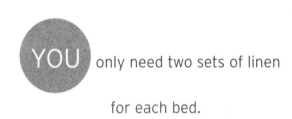 **YOU** only need two sets of linen for each bed.

GO through your personal phone

book and cross out the names of

people whom you no longer call.

TAKE all the recipes you've clipped from newspapers and maga-zines over the years and place them in a ring-binder style photo album with plastic-coated pages.

MOST catalogs and newspapers

are available online. You don't have

to clutter your house with them.

DEVELOP a tradition with your kids. Every year before their birthday and again before Christmas or Chanukah, have your children go through their toys and games and make a pile of what they're ready to give away.

PRIORITIZE.

ANY clothing that you haven't

worn for two seasons should go

either into the trash, to Goodwill, to

a friend, or to the local thrift shop.

If it's broken get it fixed

or throw it away.

ALPHABETIZE your CD

or book collection.

CLOSE THE DOOR.

You have a right to simply close the

door and forget about whatever

kind of mess is behind it.

Relax in and enjoy your own home.

IF you're still trying to live your life in a way that will please your mom, your dad, your spouse, Santa, or the powers that be, stop and ask yourself why.

KEEP a good, large pair of

scissors in the kitchen.

IT'S EASIER to handle hot

cupcake/muffin tins if you leave one

of the corners empty.

WHEN you finish a box of tissues, put the empty box on a kitchen counter and stuff it with flimsy plastic grocery bags. Once you have a full box of bags, keep it in the trunk of your car.

THINK

about your cooking
style and equip
your kitchen
accordingly.

RETHINK stereotypical roles.

It makes no sense to expend energy

doing things you're neither good at

nor enjoy, simply because those are

things that men or women are sup-

posed to do.

CREATE a kitchen bulletin

board to tack up "must-have" items

. . . such as permission slips, bills to

pay, notes to answer, and so on.

PUT your dish drainer and sponges into the dishwasher to get them really clean.

YOUR fridge and freezer are most efficient if you keep them two-thirds full, if the freezer temperature is 0°F, and if the refrigerator temperature is 37°F.

IF YOU CAN trace a nasty

kitchen odor to your garbage dis-

posal, try tossing in a lemon and

some oranges.

RATHER than scrubbing the grease-caked metal filter above your stove, place it in the dishwasher.

There should be less talk; a preaching point is not a meeting point. What do you do then? Take a broom and clean someone's house. That says enough.

MOTHER TERESA (1910–1997)

If you want to make dried herbs taste fresh, chop up an equal amount of parsley and add it to the herbs. The moisture and chlorophyll

WORK LIKE MAGIC.

TREAT yourself

to really good coffee.

WHEN you go to the trouble of making pancakes and waffles, make a few extra and freeze them in a zip-lock bag. Next time you want one, just pop it in the toaster.

DEVELOP a basic list of what

you need to have on hand for your

family.

KEEP your shopping list on your

fridge door and let everyone note

down what's missing as they eat

your cupboards bare.

Avoid shopping for dinner on your

way home from work.

Make sure your refrigerator has things in it that everyone will eat.

DEVELOP a repertoire of at

least five meals that you can pre-

pare in less than thirty minutes.

LISTENING to music is a

great and satisfying simple pleasure.

Let it be your dessert at the end of

an otherwise bland, humdrum day.

AVOID planning a meal in which

everything requires elaborate

preparation.

Never confuse movement with action.

KEEP A FEW
PREPARED MEALS IN
YOUR FREEZER.

Decide on eight or ten basic meals

that you like and always keep the

ingredients for them on hand.

WHEN you're really feeling in

the mood to cook, double the

recipes and freeze the extras.

TAKE OUT a tablecloth, cloth
napkins, your good dishes, and a
couple of candles and make dinner
look special . . . for no reason at all.

HANG your car and house keys

on a hook on your kitchen wall as

soon as you come into the house.

GIVE each member of your family

a basket for mittens, gloves, hats,

and scarves near the door.

CREATE a stationery drawer

containing paper, stamped

envelopes, address book, pens, and

a book of stamps.

Keep a duplicate
of your address
book in a safe,
fireproof box.

BUY several pairs of scissors,

pencils and pens, and rolls of tape

and sprinkle them around the house

in baskets or drawers.

STORE YOUR SHOES

in the boxes they came in.

And yet a little tumult, now and then,
is an agreeable quickener of sensation;
such as a revolution, a battle, or an
adventure of any lively description.

LORD BYRON (1788–1824)

FILL your child's closet with lots

of shelves and cubbies rather than a

hanging rod.

Keep linens on a shelf in the closet

of the room in which they're used.

KEEP a file for each pet. It's the

place to store all their medical files,

including records of vaccinations,

weight, birth history, and so on.

THINK ABOUT house-
cleaning tasks in terms of four cate-
gories: What needs to be done every
day, what needs to be done every
week, what needs to be done every
month, and what needs to be done
once or twice a year.

IF you have chores to do in more than one area of your home, plan out a route so that you don't end up retracing your steps.

ORGANIZE your cleaning

supplies in baskets. Keep a basket in

each strategic area throughout the

house.

DO your most loathsome chores first.

Simplicity of life, even the barest, is not a misery, but the very foundation of refinement; a sanded floor and white-washed walls and the green trees, and flowery meads, and living waters outside; or a grimy palace amid the same with a regiment of house-maids always working to smear the dirt together so that it may be unnoticed; which, think you, is the most refined, the most fit for a gentleman of those two dwellings?

WILLIAM MORRIS (1834–1896)

IF you live in a two-story house,

keep a vacuum on each level.

WAIT for the sun to go down to

wash your windows. This avoids

streaking.

IF your children have laundry baskets in their rooms, they can keep track of (and even do) their own laundry.

DECIDE to buy your child one

color of socks only.

IF you use cloth napkins, get a different napkin ring for each member of the family.

Dry your laundry
outside in the sun.

If you're designing or remodeling a

house, put the laundry somewhere

upstairs near the bedrooms.

Change the wallpaper or paint color

of a little-used room in your house.

KEEP a file card for each room

of your house and write down the

paint brand and color formula for

the walls, ceiling, and woodwork.

COAT your snow shovel blade

with floor wax before you start

shoveling. You won't have to knock

the snow off.

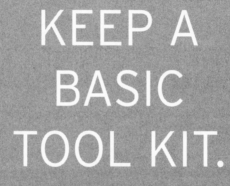

KEEP A
BASIC
TOOL KIT.

PUNCH holes in the manuals

that come with your fridge, stove,

microwave, TV, and so on, and keep

them in a ringed binder.

TO PREVENT the back of what you're drilling through from splintering, put a scrap of any kind of wood (composite board, plywood, etc.) behind it.

IF there's a tiny hole in your screen, try dabbing it with some clear nail polish.

DIP the wooden handles of your favorite garden tools into a pail of bright-colored paint. You'll be able to find your tools wherever you drop them.

Invest in really good garden tools

and take good care of them.

CARRY a
recent photo of
your child in your
car or wallet.

SIT DOWN with your family

and talk about what to do if there's

a fire or other emergency.

If you ride a bicycle, carry your

name, address, and phone number

in a seat pack. In case of a fall and

loss of consciousness, witnesses

CAN HELP.

KEEP A LIST of emergency

numbers taped onto the receiver of

each phone in your home.

REMEMBER, it isn't worth

economizing on locks.

KEEP A FLASHLIGHT,

pillow, blanket, and extra pair of

socks and gloves in the trunk of

your car.

Know how (and when) to do the

Heimlich maneuver.

Learn your blood type and make a

note of it on your driver's license.

Photocopy all of your credit cards

and put them in a safe place.

If your dog drools all over the car,

help him overcome the anxiety by

just getting in the car and having a

cozy time, without actually driving

anywhere.

USE
CRUISE
CONTROL.

An ounce of action is worth a ton of theory.

FRIEDRICH ENGELS (1820-1895)

KEEP a little bottle of touch-up

paint from your car dealer for nicks

and scratches.

TEACH your children how to

prepare a basic meal and how to do

the laundry before they reach the

age of ten.

Practice saying no.

*The greatest discovery of my genera-
tion is that a human being can alter his
life by altering his attitudes of mind.*

WILLIAM JAMES (1842–1910)

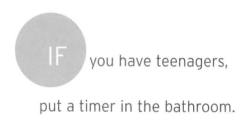 you have teenagers,

put a timer in the bathroom.

KEEP a file for each of your children. It's a place to put report cards, special drawings, newspaper clippings, and any other of the very select things you decide to save.

Keep a folder for those PAPERS that contain phone numbers or statements about school policy that might come into question over the course of the year, and NOTICES of school events. Keep the folder near the table or desk where your child unloads his/her backpack each day, and go through it at least once a week to KEEP IT CURRENT.

EVEN young children can learn

how to file and organize things, and

it's a lesson that will serve them

well as they get older.

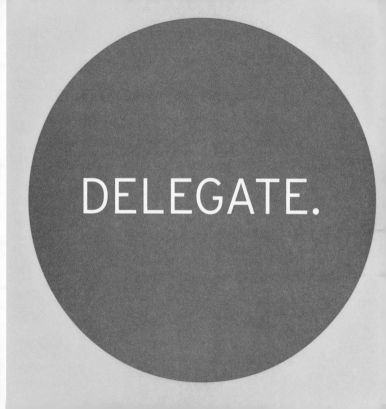

DELEGATE.

He who can take no great interest in what is small will take false interest in what is great.

JOHN RUSKIN (1819–1900)

DON'T KEEP toys in a toy

box. Use simple wooden shelves,

clear plastic storage bins, or cubbies.

IF YOU'VE GOT A

teenager who doesn't always check

in, invest in a cell phone.

SPEND the most time on the

activities that give you the greatest

pleasure or satisfaction.

Invest in an extra pair of eyeglasses.

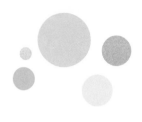

Keep a large cosmetic case, already

packed with everything you need.

ALWAYS PACK A
NIGHTLIGHT.

Schedule a regular family meeting

every Sunday evening.

Help your kids with their homework. It's worth every minute.

If you have a craving for

something . . . SATISFY IT!

TIME FLIES . . . whether

you're having fun or not.

BUY spices in bulk. They are

fresher and much less expensive.

SAVE money on a new car by

deciding to purchase it at the end of

the year when dealers are most

eager to get rid of inventory.

KEEP an inexpensive disposable

camera in your car.

FILL your gas tank when it is

only half full.

AS you pack your suitcase make a list of everything that goes in it. Keep a copy of the list at home along with a copy of your passport and itinerary. In case of theft you'll have an easier time with your insurance company.

Everything should be made as simple as possible, but not simpler.

ALBERT EINSTEIN (1879-1955)